REFLEXOLOGY

REALLY

WORKS

The Absolute Beginners Guide

BY

Mercedes Del Rey

REFLEXOLOGY REALLY WORKS by Mercedes Del Rey

REFLEXOLOGY REALLY WORKS by Mercedes Del Rey

Terms and Conditions
LEGAL NOTICE
(02052016)

The Publisher has strived to be as accurate and complete as possible in the creation of this report, notwithstanding the fact that he does not warrant or represent at any time that the contents within are accurate due to the rapidly changing nature of the Internet.

While all attempts have been made to verify information provided in this publication, the Publisher assumes no responsibility for errors, omissions, or contrary interpretation of the subject Matter herein. Any perceived slights of specific persons, peoples, or organizations are unintentional.

In practical advice books, like anything else in life, there are no guarantees of income made. Readers are cautioned to reply on their own judgment about their individual circumstances to act accordingly.

REFLEXOLOGY REALLY WORKS by Mercedes Del Rey

FREE GIFT FROM THE PUBLISHER

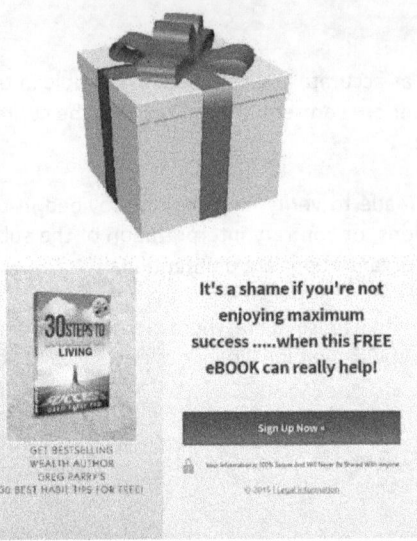

Please search this page over the internet http://www.onelifeblog.com/free-success-guide

REFLEXOLOGY REALLY WORKS by Mercedes Del Rey

Table of Contents

History of Reflexology 7

Foreword 10

Chapter 1: 13

    The Basics On Reflexology 13

    The Basics 13

FAQ 14

Chapter 2: 15

    Reflexology Points And Areas 15

    The Areas 18

Chapter 3: 19

    Assisting The Cardiovascular System 19

    The Heart 19

Chapter 4: 21

    Assisting Kidney Function 21

    About The Toxins 22

Chapter 5: 23

    Help With PMS 23

    For Women 23

Chapter 6: 25

    Bettering Quality Of Life For Cancer Patients 25

    Some Relief 25

Chapter 7: 27

    Increasing Energy and Feelings Of Wellbeing 27

    Step Up Your Vigor 27

Chapter 8: 29

    Emotional Healing With Reflexology 29

REFLEXOLOGY REALLY WORKS by Mercedes Del Rey

    The Mind 29

Chapter 9: 31

    Boosting Your Immune System 31

    The Whole Body 31

Chapter 10: 33

    How To Do Reflexology 33

    STEP BY STEP INSTRUCTIONS FOR FOOT REFLEXOLOGY! 33

CHAPTER 11 47

    How To Do Self Reflexology, Find A Practitioner And Possible Side Effects 47

    Synopsis 47

    The Inside Info 48

Wrapping Up 48

Chapter 1 51

    How to Get the Maximum Benefits from Your Workbook 51

Chapter 2 55

    Introduction to the Concept of Mindful Relaxation 55

Chapter 3 63

    How You React to Stress 63

Chapter 4 67

    Your Stress Symptoms Checklist 67

REFLEXOLOGY REALLY WORKS by Mercedes Del Rey

History of Reflexology

Modern reflexology is based on an ancient form of therapy. There is evidence of some form of foot and hand therapy being Practised in China as long ago as 4,000 B.C. and also at the same time in Egypt, as depicted in the tomb of Ankmahor. The North American tribes of Indians are known to have Practised a form of foot therapy for hundreds of years.

There is some confusion about the true origin of this powerful therapy, sufficient to say that it has stood the test of time and has helped thousands of people to better health.

The dictionary definition of a "Reflex" is "an involuntary or instinctive movement in response to a stimulus" or in the sense of reflection or mirror image.

The reflexes on our feet and hands act as mirror images of the body.

Zone Therapy was used as far back as AD1500. The American president, James Abram Garfield was said to apply pressure to his feet to relieve pain.

During the 16th Century a number of books were published on Zone Therapy, one was written by Dr Adamus and Dr A'tatis and another by Dr Ball in Leipzig.

The re-discovery of some form of systemized foot treatment is accredited to Dr. William Fitzgerald who called it Zone Therapy and drew it to the attention of the medical world between 1915 and 1917. It was in 1915 that an article entitled "To stop that toothache, squeeze your toe" was published in "Everybody's Magazine", written by Edwin Bowers, which first brought Dr. Fitzgerald's work on Zone Therapy before the public.

In 1917, Dr. Fitzgerald wrote "Zone Therapy or Relieving Pain in the Home". Two years later, they enlarged this book and published it under a second title "Zone Therapy or Curing Pain and Disease".

Dr. William Fitzgerald (1872 – 1942) received his medical degree from the University of Vermont in 1895. He practiced in Boston City Hospital for two and a half years before going to London. He spent two years at the Central London Nose and Throat hospital before taking up a position in Vienna as Assistant to Professors Politzer and Chiari, who were highly respected doctors.

Dr. Ada Politzer (1835 – 1920) of the University of Vienna, was a well-known author of many medical books and made clinical contributions to the diagnosis and treatment of diseases of the ear. Dr. Otto

REFLEXOLOGY REALLY WORKS by Mercedes Del Rey

Chiari, again an established authority, wrote several books on diseases and surgery of the larynx and trachea.

Dr Fitzgerald never published the original sources for his own therapy, but it is likely that he was influenced during this time in Vienna, by the work of Dr. d'Arsonval. In "Zone Therapy is Scientific" by Dr W D Chesney, it is stated that in Germany, Dr. d'Arsonval was using physiotherapy and getting relief following the use of reflex knowledge which, in effect, was what was later termed Zone Therapy by Drs Fitzgerald and Bowers.

When Dr Fitzgerald returned to the United States, he became head of the Nose and Throat Department at St Francis Hospital, Hartford, Connecticut. Around 1909, Dr Fitzgerald discovered, or re-discovered Zone Therapy. Almost ten years later, he wrote his book, about how he had stumbled upon the concept of Zone Therapy:

"Six years ago I accidentally discovered that pressure with a cotton tipped probe on the muco-cutinous margin (where the skin joins the mucous membrane) of the nose gave an anaesthetic result as though a cocaine solution had been applied. I further found that there were many spots in the nose, mouth, throat and on both surfaces of the tongue, which, when pressed firmly, deadened definite areas of sensation. Also, that pressure exerted over any bony eminence of the hands, feet or over the joints, produces the same characteristic results in pain relief. I found also that when pain was relieved, the condition that produced the pain was most generally relieved. This led to my 'mapping out' these various areas and their associated connections and also to noting the conditions influenced through them. This science I have named "Zone Therapy".

It is worth noting that the Chinese had, in acupuncture, divided the body into longitudinal meridians by approximately 2,500 B.C.

From 1915 and into the early 1930's, the subject of zone therapy was controversial, although it met with a certain amount of success with osteopaths and dentists.

One physician who did believe in Fitzgerald's work was Dr. Joe Shelby Riley of Washington. He and his wife, Elizabeth, credit Dr. Fitzgerald as one who, in modern times, brought this science (ie. Zone therapy) to the notice of the public.

The physiotherapist working with Dr. Riley at St Petersburg, was Eunice Ingham (1889 – 1974). Eunice Ingham extended the work of Dr. Fitzgerald and painstakingly mapped the feet with all the corresponding organs and glands of the body. She was a real pioneer who was determined to help people to help themselves, if their doctor was not using reflexology. In the early years, she worked with doctors to prove her findings and to demonstrate to them that reflexology was a useful diagnostic tool.

REFLEXOLOGY REALLY WORKS by Mercedes Del Rey

She lectured at a medical clinic headed by Dr. Charles Epstein in May 1939. In his report, he acknowledged that reflexology worked. However, while they knew it worked, doctors were not interested in using it, because reflexology was too time consuming and they could not make as much money.

Eunice Ingham is still known as the pioneer of modern reflexology and she authored two well-known books "Stories the Feet Can Tell" and "Stories the Feet Have Told". They have since been combined into one volume. In addition to her writing and lecturing, she, along with her nephew, Dwight Byers, founded the International Institute so that her work could be continued in perpetuity.

Dwight Byers is the current President of the Institute. He worked for many years with his Aunt and is equally keen that her work and that developed by the Institute more recently, should be passed on for the benefit of many people.

Throughout her forty years of experience treating many thousands of people, Eunice Ingham devised a system of techniques which enable the practitioner to contact the reflexes in the most effective and economic way. This system is known as the "Original Ingham Method" and though this method has been refined still further through research by Dwight Byers and staff at the Institute, her legacy is still thoroughly entwined in the practical techniques that we teach.

The years of World War II interrupted Eunice Ingham's travelling for a time, but in 1947 she was joined on her lecture tour by her nephew. Each of Eunice Ingham's seminars was unique. Her method of instruction was to demonstrate and lecture as she worked on the health problems of those who attended. Over the years, Dwight Byers has contributed to his aunt's work by organizing the seminars into training workshops. These have been further developed to produce the Diploma course that we teach in the UK.

Eunice Ingham died in 1974, having devoted forty years of her life to reflexology. Today, her legacy continues and she would be proud to see how reflexology has been developed into a profession. So those of us associated with the International Institute of Reflexology are indeed fortunate that we have the opportunity to get so close to the originator of the techniques.

Reflexology can benefit people of all ages and, depending on the length of time a condition has been present, can improve or eliminate many ailments during a course of four to six weekly treatments.

REFLEXOLOGY REALLY WORKS by Mercedes Del Rey

Foreword

Reflexology may be defined as a practice of applying pressure to the feet and hands using thumb, finger, and hand techniques without the use of oils, creams, or lotions. Based on a system of zones, that reflects an image of the body on the feet and hands which in turn effects the physical changes made in the body.

Definition

Reflexology is a therapeutic method of relieving pain by stimulating predefined pressure points on the feet and hands. This controlled pressure alleviates the source of the discomfort. In the absence of any particular malady or abnormality, reflexology may be as effective for promoting good health and for preventing illness as it may be for relieving symptoms of stress, injury, and illness.

Reflexologists work from maps of predefined pressure points that are located on the hands and feet. These pressure points are reputed to connect directly through the nervous system and affect the bodily organs and glands. The reflexologist manipulates the pressure points according to specific techniques of reflexology therapy. By means of this touching therapy, any part of the body that is the source of pain, illness, or potential debility can be strengthened through the application of pressure at the respective foot or hand location.

Purpose

Reflexology promotes healing by stimulating the nerves in the body and encouraging the flow of blood. In the process, reflexology not only quells the sensation of pain, but relieves the source of the pain as well.

Anecdotally, reflexologists claim success in the treatment of a variety of conditions and injuries. One condition is fibromyalgia. People with this disease are encouraged to undergo reflexology therapy to alleviate any of a number of chronic bowel syndromes associated with the condition. Frequent brief sessions of reflexology therapy are also recommended as an alternative to drug therapy for controlling the muscle pain associated with fibromyalgia and for relieving difficult breathing caused by tightness in the muscles of the patient's neck and throat.

Reflexology applied properly can alleviate allergy symptoms, as well as stress, back pain, and chronic fatigue. The techniques of reflexology can be performed conveniently on the hand in situations where a session on the feet is not practical, although the effectiveness of limited hand therapy is less

REFLEXOLOGY REALLY WORKS by Mercedes Del Rey

pronounced than with the foot pressure therapy.

Description

Origins

Reflexology is a healing art of ancient origin. Although its origins are not well documented, there are reliefs on the walls of a Sixth Dynasty Egyptian tomb (c. 2450 B.C.) that depict two seated men receiving massage on their hands and feet. From Egypt, the practice may have entered the Western world during the conquests of the Roman Empire. The concepts of reflexology have also been traced to pre-dynastic China (possibly as early as 3000 B.C.) and to ancient Indian medicine. The Inca civilization may have subscribed to the theories of reflexology and passed on the practice of this treatment to the Native Americans in the territories that eventually entered the United States.

In recent times, Sir Henry Head first investigated the concepts underlying reflexology in England in the 1890s. Therapists in Germany and Russia were researching similar notions at approximately the same time, although with a different focus. Less than two decades later, a physician named William H. Fitzgerald presented a similar concept that he called zone analgesia or zone therapy. Fitzgerald's zone analgesia was a method of relieving pain through the application of pressure to specific locations throughout the entire body. Fitzgerald divided the body into 10 vertical zones, five on each side, that extended from the head to the fingertips and toes, and from front to back. Every aspect of the human body appears in one of these 10 zones, and each zone has a reflex area on the hands and feet. Fitzgerald and his colleague, Dr. Edwin Bowers, demonstrated that by applying pressure on one area of the body, they could anesthetize or reduce pain in a corresponding part. In 1917, Fitzgerald and Bowers published Relieving Pain at Home, an explanation of zone therapy.

Later, in the 1930s, a physical therapist, Eunice D. Ingham, explored the direction of the therapy and made the startling discovery that pressure points on the human foot were situated in a mirror image of the corresponding organs of the body with which the respective pressure points were associated. Ingham documented her findings, which formed the basis of reflexology, in Stories the Feet Can Tell, published in 1938. Although Ingham's work in reflexology was inaccurately described as zone therapy by some, there are differences between the two therapies of pressure analgesia. Among the more marked differences, reflexology defines a precise correlation between pressure points and afflicted areas of the body. Furthermore, Ingham divided each foot and hand into 12 respective pressure zones, in contrast to the 10 vertical divisions that encompass the entire body in Fitzgerald's zone therapy.

In 1968 two siblings, Dwight Byers and Eusebia Messenger, established the National Institute of

REFLEXOLOGY REALLY WORKS by Mercedes Del Rey

Reflexology. By the early 1970s the institute had grown and was renamed the International Institute of Reflexology.

In a typical reflexology treatment, the therapist and patient have a preliminary discussion prior to therapy, to enable the therapist to focus more accurately on the patient's specific complaints and to determine the appropriate pressure points for treatment.

A reflexology session involves pressure treatment that is most commonly administered in foot therapy sessions of approximately 40-45 minutes in duration. The foot therapy may be followed by a brief 15-minute hand therapy session. No artificial devices or special equipment are associated with this therapy. The human hand is the primary tool used in reflexology. The therapist applies controlled pressure with the thumb and forefinger, generally working toward the heel of the foot or the outer palm of the hand. Most reflexologists apply pressure with their thumbs bent; however, some also use simple implements, such as the eraser end of a pencil. Reflexology therapy is not massage, and it is not a substitute for medical treatment.

Reflexology is a complex system that identifies and addresses the mass of 7,000 nerve endings that are contained in the foot. Additional reflexology addresses the nerves that are located in the hand. This is a completely natural therapy that affords relief without the use of drugs. The Reflexology Association of America (RAA) formally discourages the use of oils or other preparations in performing this hands-on therapy.

Preparations

In order to realize maximum benefit from a reflexology session, the therapist as well as the patient should be situated so as to afford optimal comfort for both. Patients in general receive treatment in a reclining position, with the therapist positioned as necessary—to work on the bare feet, or alternately on the bare hands.

A reflexology patient removes both shoes and socks in order to receive treatment. No other preparation is involved. No prescription drugs, creams, oils, or lotions are used on the skin.

Precautions

Reflexology is extremely safe. It may even be self-administered in a limited form whenever desired. The qualified reflexologist offers a clear and open disclaimer that reflexology does not constitute medical treatment in any form, nor is reflexology given as a substitute for medical advice or treatment. The ultimate purpose of the therapy is to promote wellness; fundamentally it is a form of preventive therapy.

REFLEXOLOGY REALLY WORKS by Mercedes Del Rey

Chapter 1:

The Basics On Reflexology

Synopsis

This is a popular form of detecting and addressing any possible ailments, illnesses, or diseases the body may be undergoing. In ancient times this method was used to ensure that any possible negative problems in the body are arrested before it progresses to a point where it would be difficult to treat.

The Basics

Using reflexology to restore the equilibrium balance by means of the foot or hand is a rather strange but totally accurate. Many people have tried reflexology to address specific medical problems with overwhelmingly successful results.

The pressure sensors in the feet and hands are all connected to various parts of the body's systems. It functions like a network of intricate connections flowing from one to the other. By using reflexology, the experienced practitioner is able to pinpoint the cause of the problem and manipulate it through a succession of pressure points on the feet or palms of the hands. All these sensors work and respond to the sometimes light but mostly painful pressures on the feet and hands.

Other deviations but equally suitable forms of reflexology are walking on a pebble path, using foot massages that simulate reflexology movements, and using rollers. Surprisingly other simple tools like a golf ball can also be used as reflexology item though they are not as good as the original natural way of the thumb and finger.

Reflexology sessions ideally last for bout 30 – 45 minutes, as any longer might cause undue stress to the already pain heightened situation. The reflexologist uses pressure, stretches and movements to work thought the foot methodically. After which an assessment on the body condition may be given.

REFLEXOLOGY REALLY WORKS by Mercedes Del Rey

FAQ

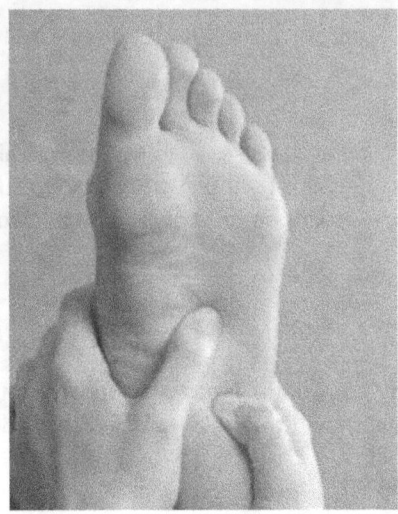

Is Reflexology safe?

Yes. Practitioners trained in the Original Ingham Method of Reflexology have the knowledge and skills to work with people of all ages, from newborn babies to the elderly, including the provision of professional reflexology during pregnancy, chemotherapy and palliative care.

Is Reflexology painful?

Reflexology can be extremely relaxing, however if there is a part of the body that is unbalanced, the corresponding reflex point may feel sore or tender whilst the practitioner works to rebalance the area. If at any time you find the treatment painful, please tell your Practitioner, as it is important that they work within your comfort-zone.

Is Reflexology ticklish?

No. The way in which a professional Reflexologist holds and works the feet is with a firm pressure which is not at all ticklish.

REFLEXOLOGY REALLY WORKS by Mercedes Del Rey

Chapter 2:

Reflexology Points And Areas

Synopsis

Ideally the chart on the subject on reflexology reflects the various pressure points and their corresponding parts of the different organs, glands, structures, and systems of the anatomy. These charts can also be looked upon as maps of the intricate workings of the human body.

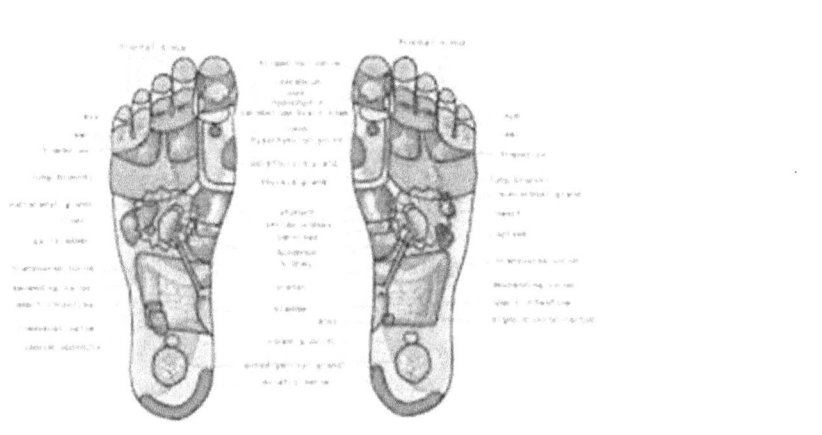

REFLEXOLOGY REALLY WORKS by Mercedes Del Rey

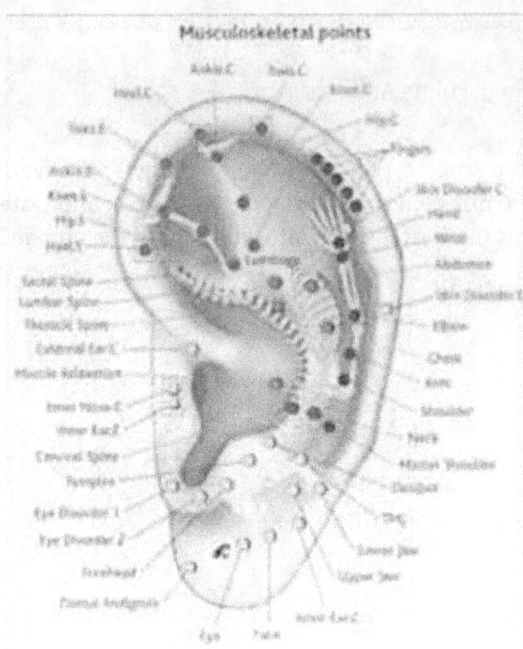

REFLEXOLOGY REALLY WORKS by Mercedes Del Rey

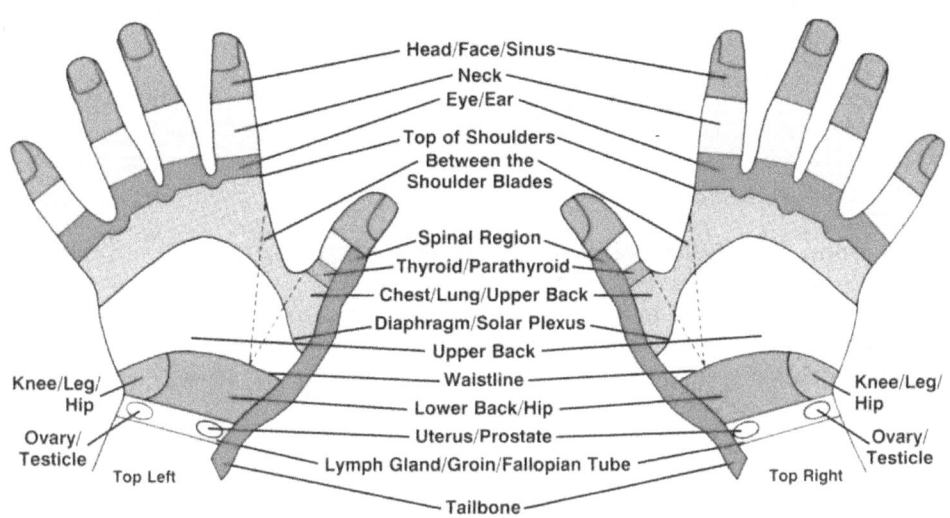

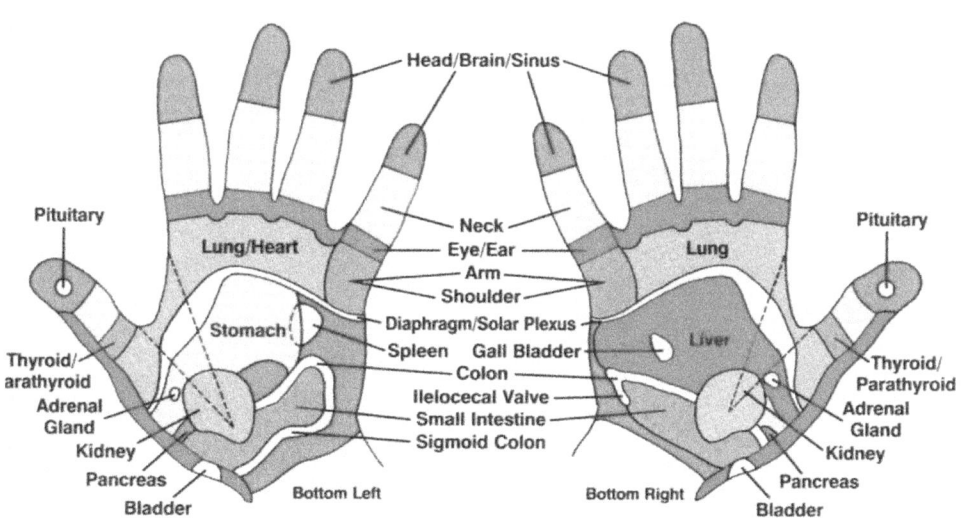

REFLEXOLOGY REALLY WORKS by Mercedes Del Rey

The Areas

Though popularly accepted as a foot and hand, palm focused style of treatment; there are also instances of having the reflexology points in the ear area. Simply put, reflexology sessions strive to open up the stubble energy channels thus directing reflexology pressure points to stimulation mode.

The ear also has various pressure points which are connected to the autonomic functions of the heart and stomach. When addressed these pressure points seem to successfully invoke stronger autonomic responses in the cardiac and gastric systems when compared to the foot or palms. The ear lobes seem to contain master sensory points which affect the eyes, pineal and pituitary glands.

According to medical research there are 10 zones or meridians that are logistically located in the human body. For instance, when pressure is applied to the big toe the benefits are seen in the brain area. Likewise, when pressure is applied to the base of the foot, it treats the neck and throat ailments. Pressure on the ball of the foot puts the connection through to the lungs and heart. The foot arch when pressed affects the adrenals, kidneys, gastrointestinal track, and bladder. The middle of the foot when pressured affects the waistline, while the ankle bone affects sexual functions.

Being supposedly easy to detect these various pressure points and their connections for treatment is not reason enough to completely discontinue an ongoing medical treatment program. Even if reflexology is considered as an added complimenting factor, a doctor's opinion should always be sought, especially if the illness is serious.

Chapter 3:

Assisting The Cardiovascular System

Synopsis

Ideally when treating a particular illness, ailment or disease, it should not be the practice to only address the particular area affected but besides focusing on the affected area, the other parts of the body should also be looked into.

The Heart

When a reflexologist treats an individual this is the primary concern. The reflexologist not only focuses on the problem but also try to ensure all the other connecting factors are addressed too. Therefore, the individual facing cardiovascular problems should expect to be treated holistically as the art of reflexology demands.

As the cardiovascular system is made up of various corresponding part, which are the heart, arteries, veins, arterioles, venules and capillaries, it should be notes that the actual heart may not be the problem area. Its purpose is to carry all the nutrients and oxygen to the various parts of the body. When these are blocked for one reason or another then reflexology is a good first address.

Using reflexology to reestablish the optimum flow and circulation in the system is a good noninvasive way of treating the problem before it escalates to a more serious level.

Using reflexology, the heart reflexes are addressed as this organ is the instrument that pumps the blood thought-out the body. Then the kidneys are the next in line to be addressed.

The kidneys filter the blood constantly. The diaphragm and chest are also noted by the reflexologist because these reflexes would be worked to encourage relaxation in the chest cavity and promote deeper breathing.

Lastly the spinal area is also checked. Located on the inner edges of the feet the spine reflexes would be stimulated to promote communication through the nervous system.
Sometimes reflexology can also be used in the case of an actual heart attack, though it is not

REFLEXOLOGY REALLY WORKS by Mercedes Del Rey

recommended if there is immediate medical response available.

Chapter 4:

Assisting Kidney Function

Synopsis

The kidneys in a human body have a vital part to play in maintaining the body at its optimum levels. This organ is responsible for eliminating all the waste and toxins from the body's circulatory system. When there is a buildup of all these negative elements the problems like renal failure may occur. Therefore, the cleansing method or condition the body should adopt to keep the negative buildups from occurring is by using reflexology.

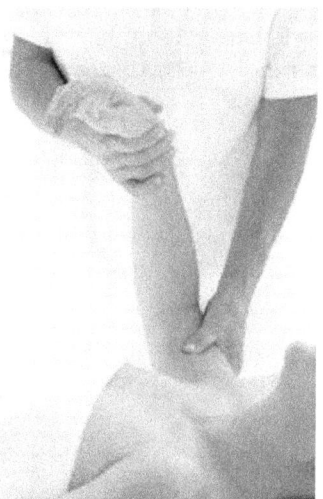

REFLEXOLOGY REALLY WORKS by Mercedes Del Rey

About The Toxins

Reflexology is a safe and proven method of addressing this, before it becomes a major problem for the body system. Making reflexology a good part of the health care regiment for an individual will help avoid any serious medical issues. Vectorial reflexology methods use very precise reflex points developed from the anatomy to eliminate any possible kidney problems.

When starting a reflexology session, the individual hand and feet should be easily accessible. The reflexology kidney zone is in the palm so by placing the individual's palm in the reflexologist hands and then applies pressure downwards between the index finger and the middle finger rub in deep movements.

After doing this for both palms, the reflexologist can now move on to the feet. By rubbing the thumbs down the foot to the bottom of the arch in-between the big toe and next to the other kidney zone is addressed. This area should be rubbed vigorously. All this is done for a reasonable period of time until the pain and discomfort disappears.

In using the reflexology exercise the intention is to create the ideal circumstance to assure the flow of energy is restored to its optimum levels again. These pressures should trigger the brain to discharge the negative direct current of regeneration in to the deficient are of the body. The intention is to help clear the interstitial space of congestive debris and bring the body to a more efficient cellular level.

REFLEXOLOGY REALLY WORKS by Mercedes Del Rey

Chapter 5:

Help With PMS

Synopsis

All women go through the time where a menstrual cycle is part of their lives. The lucky ones breeze through this time of the month comfortably while there are others who are not so lucky. They may experience symptoms like bloating, sleepless nights cravings mood swings and many others.

For Women

Reflexology has been known to be able to provide some form of relief to ease the discomfort brought on by the menstrual cycle or otherwise referred to as PMS.

Most people who sought this method to address the discomfort endured every month have been pleased with the results. The reflexologist will begin the session from a holistic point of view.

With this in mind, certain reflex parts will be emphasized as these areas are in direct correspondence to the body parts and organ being affected by the PMS condition.

The reflexologist will spend an extra amount of time on the kidney reflex are if the individual is complaining of bloating or of water retention symptoms.

The glands and organs responsible for regulating the hormones would be another area the reflexologist would focus on as this area generally affects the specific symptoms being experienced.

The areas that might be addressed are as listed below:

- The brain – this area is pin pointed because of the serotonin pathways

- Digestive system – also because of the serotonin element which can be found in the intestinal walls

REFLEXOLOGY REALLY WORKS by Mercedes Del Rey

- Central nervous system – is another reflex area

- Endocrine system reflexes

- Relaxation techniques - using reflex points this area of tension is address as it does negatively affect the PMS cycle.

Reflexology should only be sought if the PMS symptoms are fairly mild or irritatingly uncomfortable.

If the PMS symptoms are of a more severe nature other medical sources should be consulted first.

As in all things disregarding proper medical treatment in favor of alternative style treatments should only be done with the knowledge and advice of a medical physician familiar with the individual's medical condition.

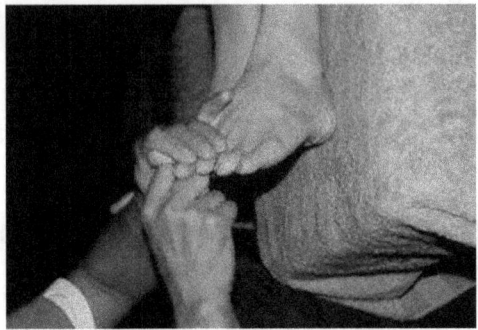

REFLEXOLOGY REALLY WORKS by Mercedes Del Rey

Chapter 6:

Bettering Quality Of Life For Cancer Patients

Synopsis

When an individual first discovers a dreaded disease like cancer is present in his or her body, the effects can be mentally devastating to say the least. Most people fall apart initially, for the lucky ones however, after absorbing the initial shock, they dive in and find out about the disease as much as possible and also all the relevant styles of medical or natural treatments that are available.

Some Relief

Reflexology has been one such discovery made. Many who use reflexology as a treatment that compliments the ongoing medical treatment have attested to being completely satisfied with the positive results. The commencement and incorporation of reflexology into the general treatment regiment, of course should only be done with a doctor's consent.

When the reflexology therapy is used to treat the patient, it is done with various intentions in mind. Some of these intentions are to provide comfort and peace of mind, to lessen the impact of side effects caused by the medical treatments, such as pain, anxiety, nausea, vomiting, fatigue, stress, depression, and fatigue. Other areas also to be addressed by reflexology are the improvements of the quality of life after chemotherapy, mood swings, quality of sleep, morale, and vital signs.

All cancer patients experience stress at various levels and at various intervals during the onset and treatment of the disease. As most negative medical conditions are somehow linked to causing more damage in the body system, reflexology can be used to correct the stress levels effectively. Reflexology is a gentle, effective tool used to assist in supporting and encouraging the patient to be in a better frame of mind and body.

By trying to create some sense of harmony in an already traumatic condition, reflexology works to play a positive role in creating a healing environment during and after the course of medical treatments.

REFLEXOLOGY REALLY WORKS by Mercedes Del Rey

REFLEXOLOGY REALLY WORKS by Mercedes Del Rey

Chapter 7:

Increasing Energy and Feelings Of Wellbeing

Synopsis

A good percentage of people today are very concerned with their health. This concern may lead them to take better care of the diet and prompt them to exercise more frequently and consistently.

However when there are medical problems, the first choice they usually make is to seek medical advice.

While this is of course a wise thing to do, some other alternatives may solve the problem better without the individual having to ingest foreign elements into the body to treat the condition.

The human body already comes with its own healing tools, but sometimes these tools just need that little help to ensure optimum successful results.

Step Up Your Vigor

One option to choose when experiencing mild medical problems is reflexology. Reflexology address the problem is a holistic manner and not just the problem itself.

All contributing factors, needs to be addressed, while detecting the root cause, and meting out the necessary pressures. As the toxins build up in our body systems, something should be done to address this condition before these said toxins begin to cause negative medical conditions. Reflexology helps to

REFLEXOLOGY REALLY WORKS by Mercedes Del Rey

ensure all the body organs are working efficiently toward this goal.

In a reputably conducted reflexology session the individual can expect to benefit holistically because there are various aspects that are addressed. These include improving the general circulation in the body system, relieving pain, and stimulated the immune and nervous systems. Each body system is addressed individually with the intention of correcting any disorders that may be present.

The blood circulation system is addressed because it contributes to the wellbeing condition of the varicose veins, hemorrhoids, and high blood pressure. In the case of the digestive system, reflexology is sought to keep the following conditions under control or eliminate them all together; stomach upsets, stomach bloating, irritable bowel syndrome, colitis, diarrhea, and ulcers. The nervous system is for addressing any possible sleep disorders, depression, and lack of concentration or energy and memory loss.

REFLEXOLOGY REALLY WORKS by Mercedes Del Rey

Chapter 8:

Emotional Healing With Reflexology

Synopsis

The most common reason people seek out reflexology sessions is to ensure their stress levels are kept under control or eliminated altogether. This is because a stress free body is a healthy body.

Even if a foot massage is given without any real reflexology techniques, the receiver would be induced into a state of relaxation and peace. The more often an individual is able to have the peace and relaxation condition within the body system, the less stress levels are detected is any at all.

The Mind

Therefore, using reflexology to control emotions is beneficial to the overall health of an individual. As reflexology is used in general to support and encourage the body to right itself, it can be a major element in controlling the emotions that are the byproduct of various negative medical conditions.

Reflexology can be used to resolve the negative emotional states brought on by anger, grief, fear, guilt, stress, jealousy, and depression.

The negative energy is released out to the individual's system using the various pressure points related to addressing this particular issue. As the meridian system is the communicator between all the various organs any physiological systems the energy flow can be sustained at an optimum level using reflexology.

The effects of emotions have a direct impact on the health condition of the body as previously pointed out. The body consists of fluids like blood, lymph, urine, sweat, semen and cerebral-spinal fluid all of which are reflected in the feet and can be recognized by a trained and experienced reflexologist.

The fluids need to be in a constant flowing motion and when they are prevented from

REFLEXOLOGY REALLY WORKS by Mercedes Del Rey

doing so, due to reasons like blockages then the problem cycle begins. Using reflexology to remove these blockages through the various pressure points is a good noninvasive excepted action.

REFLEXOLOGY REALLY WORKS by Mercedes Del Rey

Chapter 9:

Boosting Your Immune System

Synopsis

The human immune system is the first line of defense the body has for addressing potential negative elements. These elements may consist of viruses, diseases, illnesses and others. Understanding the immune system is very important to an individual's who intends to always stay healthy.

The Whole Body

Besides removing waste matter of the different forms, the immune system is responsible for protecting the body from external influences that are harmful to the body and facilitating the smooth flow of the interstitial fluids.

It also identifies all bacteria and pathogen cells and eliminates them. The immune system helps the various body parts to stay at optimum conditions in order to carry out all its particular functions successfully.

The smooth flow of the fluids can sometimes cause complications to the other functioning organs when there is a blockage. Reflexology can address this blockage of fluids properly and in a reasonable amount of time.

By listening to the bones, the reflexologist is able to tell if there are pulls in the connective tissues. If not remedied, these pulls, can affect the fluid flow patterns in the body.

Upon locating these pulls the reflexologist with then begin working on the foot, palm or ear areas to put pressure in specific points to try to relieve the area and relax the pulls until they reach their normal conditions.

Reflexology is also beneficial as a preventive measure for good health, with particular attention being paid to the immune system; the individual is able to keep the balance of the equilibrium thus aiding the body systems to work more efficiently. Regular treatments to address a specific problem, or just to ensure the body condition is in shape is a good habit to form.

If one's immune system is working efficiently then, there would be no need or a lesser need to visit the doctor so often. Also the immune system will be able to fight off any

REFLEXOLOGY REALLY WORKS by Mercedes Del Rey

outside infections more successfully.

REFLEXOLOGY REALLY WORKS by Mercedes Del Rey

Chapter 10:

How To Do Reflexology

STEP BY STEP INSTRUCTIONS FOR FOOT REFLEXOLOGY!

Start now by learning the technique you will use;

Foot Reflexology Technique

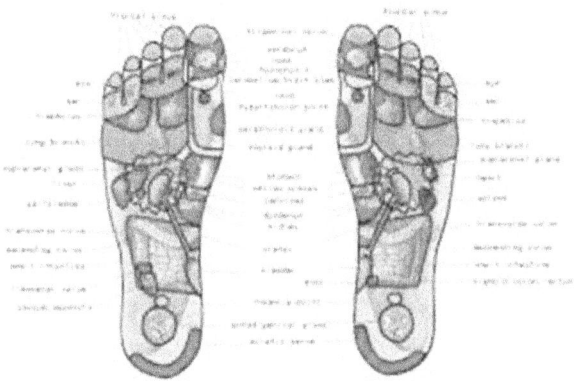

Thumb Walking

This is the most used technique for doing foot reflexology

It is easy, can be done for long periods of time without straining your hand and is extremely effective on the feet

Your thumb walks forward by itself simply by you bending and unbending the thumb.

REFLEXOLOGY REALLY WORKS by Mercedes Del Rey

Step 1.

Which part of the Thumb to use

1a. put your hands palm together in front of your face and look at the tops of your thumbs

1b. roll thumbs together at the top slightly so the nails are just touching

1c. feel the part of your thumbs where they are touching each other just on the inside at the top

This is the part of the thumb to use when thumb walking, the inside edge of the very top of your thumbs, (edge meaning that it is furthest away from the fingers of the same hand when the hand is put flat on a table)

REFLEXOLOGY REALLY WORKS by Mercedes Del Rey

Step 2.

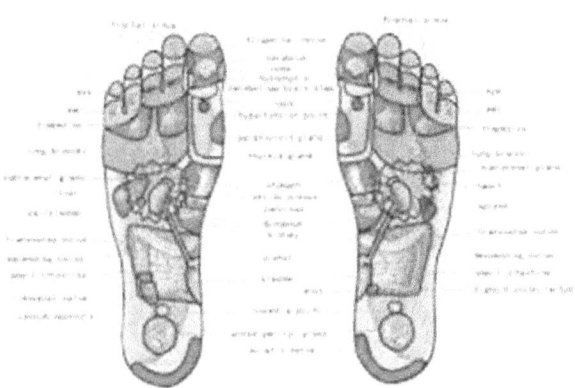

Thumb Walking Technique

2a. hold a pen with one hand (if you don't have a pen any similar surface is fine)

2b. with the other hand, put your thumb on the pen touching it with the part of the thumb described in the first step

2c. bend your thumb

2d. without moving anything else, simply straighten your thumb making sure that it stays in contact with the pen

You will notice two things

- your thumb crept slightly forward

- you are now able to apply a little bit of pressure with the part of your thumb that is touching the pen

2e. repeat; Bend, unbend, bend, unbend

REFLEXOLOGY REALLY WORKS by Mercedes Del Rey

Apply pressure at the unbend and creep forward in the bend.

Practice this technique slowly, it gets easier and faster with practice

It is easy learning foot reflexology techniques, pratically anything is a great surface to practice on; tables, chairs, TV remote controls... anything can be thumb walked!

This technique is used for the entire foot

Thumb walking allows a reflexologist to apply stimulating pressure to every single part of the foot, giving a thorough and relaxing treatment

How to do Reflexology on the Feet

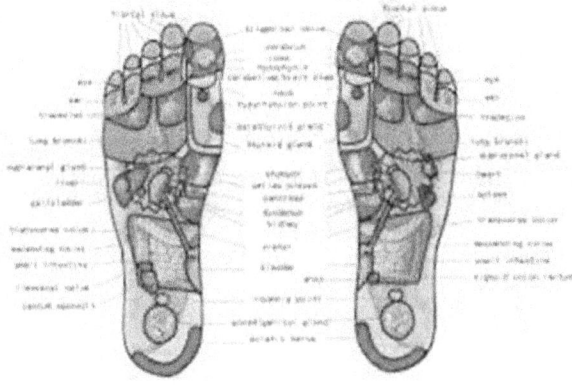

Begin every foot reflexology session on the right foot, do the whole foot, followed by the left.

Step 1.

Relaxation Exercises

REFLEXOLOGY REALLY WORKS by Mercedes Del Rey

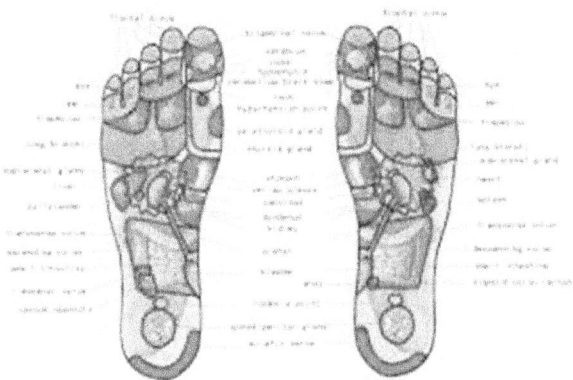

1a. massage the foot all over slowly but firmly to loosen it up, beginning at the toes moving down towards the heel, for about thirty seconds

1b. using both hands, hold on to the spine area with the palm of the hands- fingers on top of the foot and thumbs on bottom of the foot.

1c. slowly and gently twist/ wring the hands away from each other in order to gently twist the spine area on the foot. This is a relaxation exercise. Loosely wring one way and the other for about thirty seconds total

Step 2.

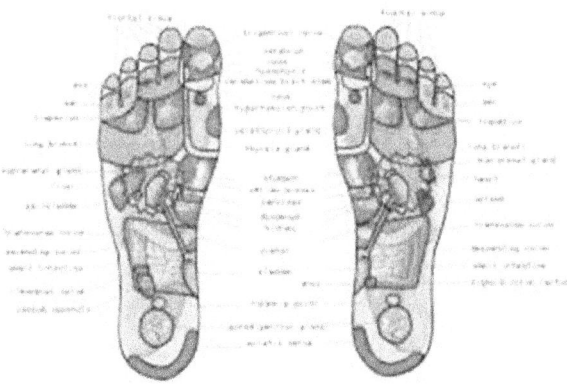

Thumb Walking the Spine

2a. thumb walk up the spine from the bottom of the heel to the tip of the big toe

REFLEXOLOGY REALLY WORKS by Mercedes Del Rey

2b. thumb walk down the spine from top of the tip of the big toe to the bottom of the heel

2c. thumb walk down the spine, but across-ways- from right to left for the entire length of the inside of the foot, see diagram below

Step 3.

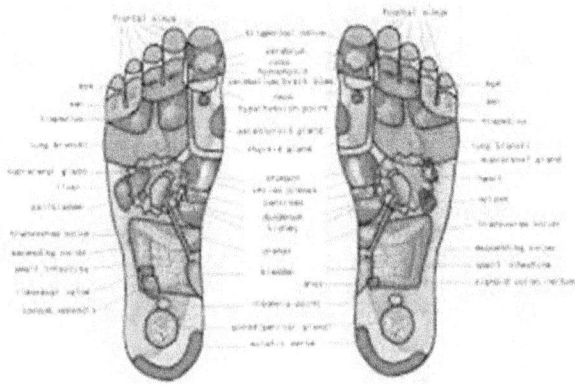

Rotate the Toes

Begin with big toe, continue toe by toe until the smallest end toe

3a. hold the toe firmly at the base of the toe, gently move in circular motions so that you are rotating and stretching the base joint that attaches the toe to the foot

3b. hold the toe just above the second joint and again move the joint in a large circular motion

3c. rotate the very top joint on the toe (the big toe only has two joints)

This foot reflexology step is great for relieving headaches as it relates to all of the bones in the skull, jaw... every bone in the head

REFLEXOLOGY REALLY WORKS by Mercedes Del Rey

When learning how to do reflexology remember the bones protecting our brain are fused together but are also separate bones, rotating the toes sends extra blood flow to their joints

Step 4.

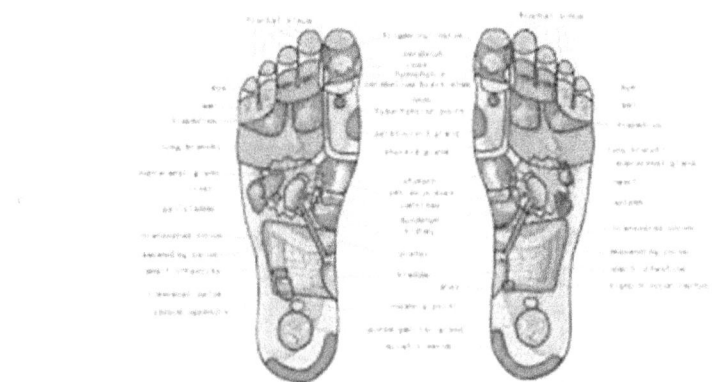

Stimulate Meridian Points on Toes

There are meridian points at the end of all the toes except the middle toe

See the diagram below for the exact points, they are easy to remember because they are pretty much under each toe nail!

4a. support the toe and use one finger to apply pressure on the meridian point in a circular motion - clockwise, then anti-clockwise, do each toe for ten seconds beginning with the big toe and finish with the little toe

Step 5.

REFLEXOLOGY REALLY WORKS by Mercedes Del Rey

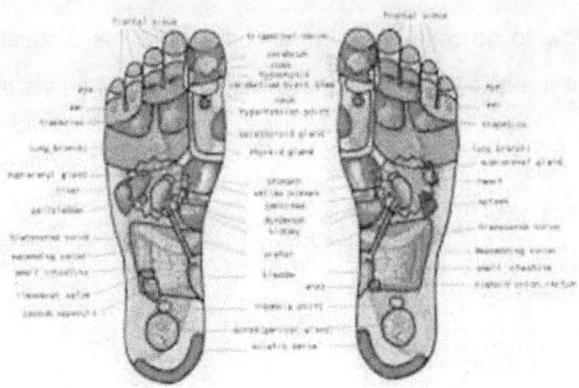

Thumb Walk the Toes

5a. thumb walk the toes in an upwards direction. Begin at the base and move upwards in a straight line to the tip.

Repeat on all sides of each toe, applying gentle but firm pressure. Begin with the big toe and finish with the little toe.

Some people like lots of pressure when thumb walking their feet, most people will not because it will stop the reflexology from being relaxing, and its supposed to be relaxing

Some peoples toes are extremely sensitive

The amount of pressure you use with any reflexology technique is relative to how much pressure the person is comfortable with, and so it is relaxing for them (although do be firm, too soft and you will tickle them!)

If there is pain in someones foot, take a break from doing reflexology on them for a while

REFLEXOLOGY REALLY WORKS by Mercedes Del Rey

Step 6.

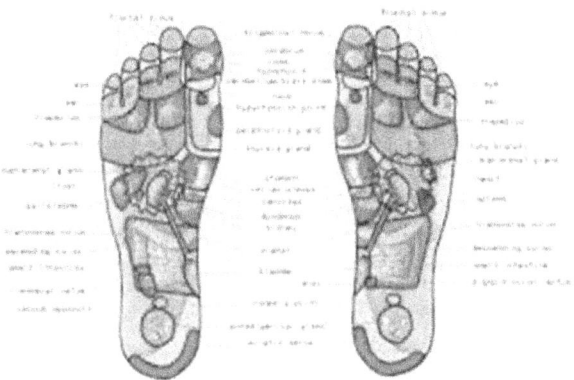

Thumb Walk Chest Area

The chest area is the ball of the foot

See exact area in foot reflexology diagram above

6a. gently thumb walk over the entire chest area in the upwards direction, then downwards and then on an angle

Step 7.

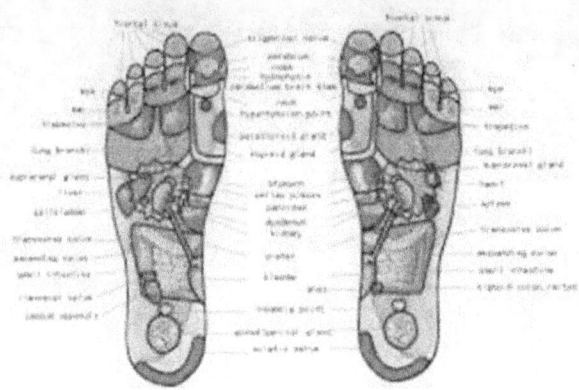

Thumb Walk Top and Back of Foot

This is a very sensitive area for most people.

7a. thumb walk from one side of the foot to the other side ie; from the toes to the ankle, for the entire top of the foot

7b. thumb walk from side to side- from right to left sides of the foot, for the entire top of the foot

REFLEXOLOGY REALLY WORKS by Mercedes Del Rey

Step 8.

Thumb Walk Liver/ Stomach area

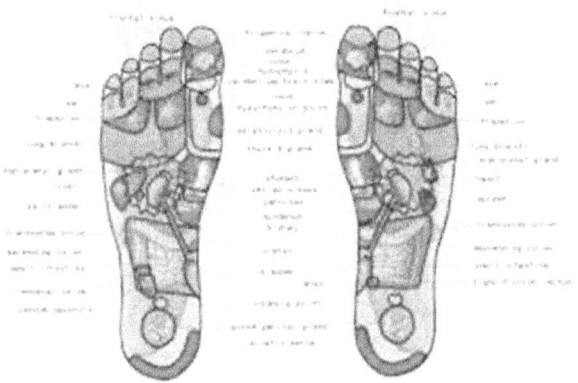

The waistline is the thinnest part of the bottom of the foot and may be further up or down and is in a different spot for everyone

Use the diagram at step six to locate the waistline

8a. thumb walk on an angle across the area between the chest area and above the waistline

8b. thumb walk on the opposite angle back across the area

This area contains the very important liver and stomach, depending on which foot you are working

Step 9.

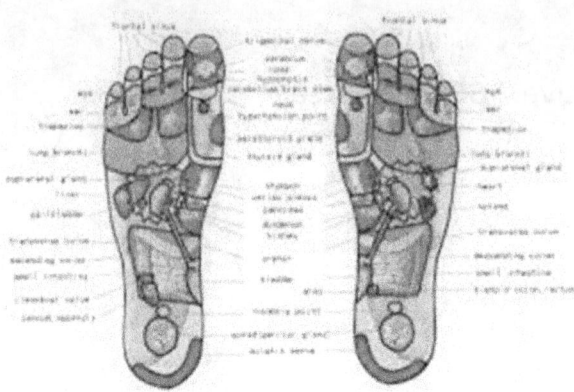

Thumb Walk Intestinal area

Use the diagram at step six to locate the waistline on the bottom of the foot

The large and small intestines are in this area

9a. thumb walk on an angle across the area between the waistline and the pelvic area

9b. thumb walk on the opposite angle back across the same area

For extra foot reflexology, check out the reflexology foot chart and see the direction that food moves through the intestines, and thumb walk in the same direction, the direction is different for the left and the right feet

Step 10.

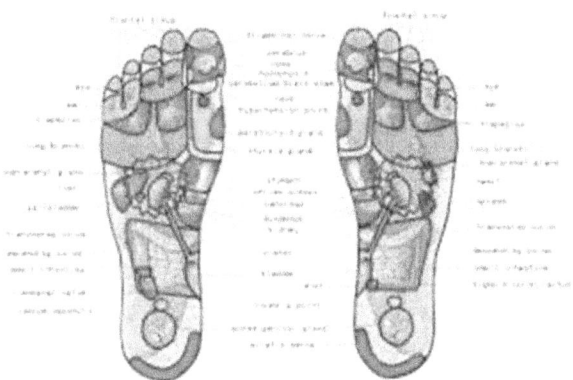

Thumb Walk Pelvic area

Use the diagram at step six to locate the pelvic area

This area relates to the Sciatic Nerve which runs up both legs

10. thumb walk from left to right over this area, go all the way up either side of the heel

10b. thumb walk the back of the heel

10c. finish reflexology with a gentle relaxing massage of the foot for one minute

Step 11.

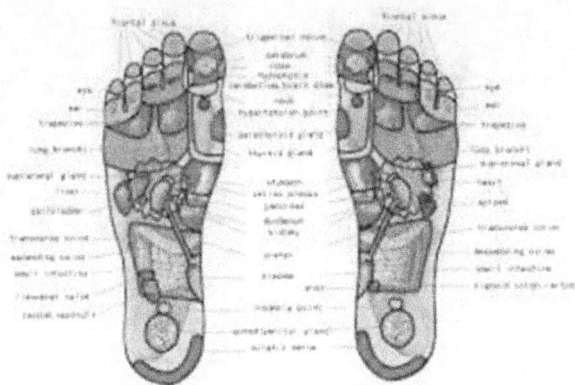

Repeat on Left Foot

11a. Go back to Step 1. and repeat each step on the left foot

REFLEXOLOGY REALLY WORKS by Mercedes Del Rey

CHAPTER 11

How To Do Self Reflexology, Find A Practitioner And Possible Side Effects

Synopsis

It is interesting to note that reflexology can be done as self help. In order to address certain specific problems a careful study of a reflexology chart must be done. Visiting a certified reflexologist for the initial consultation before embarking on the path on one's own would be better.

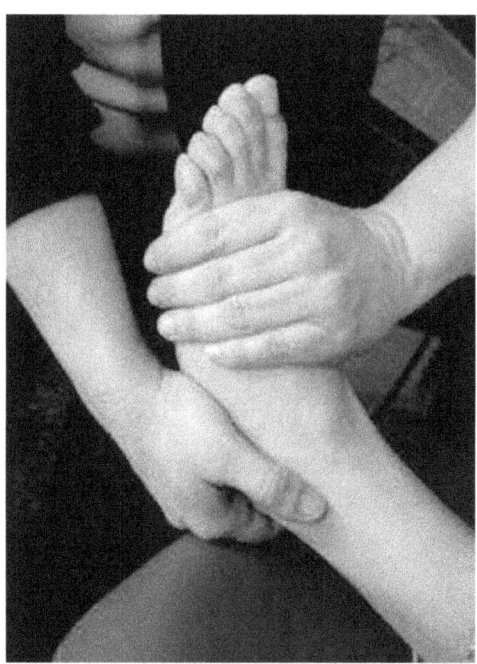

REFLEXOLOGY REALLY WORKS by Mercedes Del Rey

The Inside Info

Specific illnesses and problems are treated by targeting specific points. This can be located at the foot, palm of the hands and ears.

The easiest form of self reflexology is to follow these steps:

- While sitting comfortable bring the foot up and rest it over the opposite knee. Lace your fingers with your toes and rotate the foot at the ankle clockwise and then switch to anti-clockwise.
- Gently stretch the foot by pulling it upwards and back, all the while keeping the finger and toes laced.
- Place the ball of the foot or heel between both hands
- Placing the hands on either side of the foot gently but firmly apply pressure to each part starting with the toes, then alternate with a kneading motion.
- Forming knuckles press the first against the foot and then apply pressure going in an up and down motion.
- May finish off with a lotion rub to address any "missed" areas.

Wrapping Up

Though it may seem fairly easy to perform the reflexology moves on one's self there are some precautions that need to be taken and also some points that everyone needs to be weary off.

Certain conditions may not permit the reflexology to be done on the feet, perhaps due to the pain factor, then the exercise has to b=done on the palms of the hands.

When already ill, if reflexology is done on the feet, further toxins will be emitted into the body and this will cause a further deterioration of health.

If a fracture of broken bone condition has occurred it would be a serious folly to administer the reflexology style of treatment, as the pain involved will stress the individual further.

All in all, reflexology is safe, but always make sure to check with your doctor or reflexologist first.

REFLEXOLOGY REALLY WORKS by Mercedes Del Rey

FREE BONUS EXTRACT FROM

The MINDFUL RELAXATION BLUEPRINT

Your Personal Stress Release Workbook
Transform YOUR Life
REJUVENATE AND REGENERATE

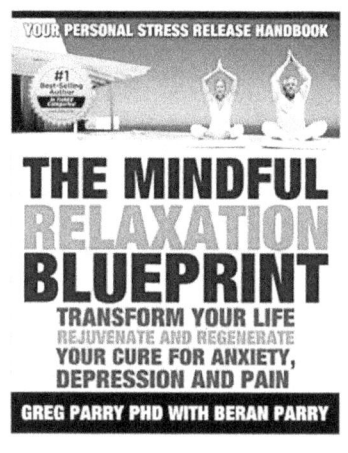

REFLEXOLOGY REALLY WORKS by Mercedes Del Rey

REFLEXOLOGY REALLY WORKS by Mercedes Del Rey

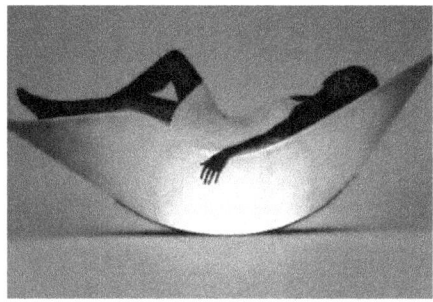

Chapter 1

How to Get the Maximum Benefits from Your Workbook

A warm welcome to your personal stress-management and mindful relaxation guide. This manual has been designed to improve your life with a series of powerful and effective relaxation techniques and mindfulness training exercises. Each technique is presented with background information followed by the appropriate, step-by-step exercises. As you practice and integrate these techniques into your daily experience, you will gain new insights into your personal stress response system and learn how to create balance and a deeper sense of well-being at every level of your life.

Simply stated, the problem today is that stress and tension have become constant factors in our lives. They're part of the background fabric of our daily experience. We need to address this problem and make a commitment to improve the quality of how we experience life every single day. Stress management and effective relaxation can only be truly effective if you choose to make them a part of your daily routine.

As you practise and assimilate the techniques in this book, you'll be able to integrate them into your repertoire of skills and gain direct access to their benefits whenever the need arises, without having to refer to the written materials.

The main benefit of regular, conscious practice is the development of great habits that will encourage you to become more naturally balanced, more centred and more relaxed all the way down to the subconscious levels where so much of our behaviour is encoded.

Here are some suggestions that will help you to maximise the benefits of relaxation on a daily basis:

- Commit to your personal programme of mindful relaxation. Make a firm agreement with yourself to set aside a specific time each day that is solely dedicated to the relaxation techniques. Write your decision on a sheet of paper and put it somewhere prominent to remind you of your pledge. It might sound simple but you'll feel better as soon as you've made that written commitment on that sheet of paper.

- The length of time required to practice the relaxation techniques each day will depend on the characteristics of each individual technique. Start gently on a modest scale. Performing a relaxation exercise for five minutes a day will yield better results than doing it only once a week for an hour. Aim for twenty to thirty minutes of relaxation

REFLEXOLOGY REALLY WORKS by Mercedes Del Rey

time once or twice a day. This is a guideline. Much will depend initially on the intensity and frequency of the day's challenges!

- You'll be able to work out the best time to relax every day by answering these two simple questions: When do you need to relax most? When can you realistically take a break from the demands of the day to make some much-needed time for yourself?

Here are some examples of how students in our relaxation and awareness classes have typically planned their activities:

- Pledge to start the day as you wake up with a calming, stabilising, relaxation exercise to help you become more focused and creative in dealing with the potentially stressful demands of the day.

- Schedule a short relaxation break during the day to neutralise habitual tensions that could result in painful physical reactions such as headaches or indigestion.

- Plan for a refreshing mid-afternoon nap to restore mental functioning and tone down the day's tiring old stress response

- Pause and relax before leaving work or arriving at home to release the tensions of the day and cultivate a calming, re-energising sense of wellbeing in the comfort of your own home.

- Practise relaxation exercises before going to sleep to promote deeply restorative rest and boost the probability of waking up feeling completely refreshed.

IN ADDITION….

- Find a quiet place to practise the techniques where you won't be interrupted. Once assimilated, many of the relaxation methods described in this workbook can be performed whenever you find yourself in a stressful or potentially difficult situation.
- Since this is probably a new activity for you, it's a good idea to let the people around you know what you're doing. Ask for their help and support by respecting your need to be alone for short periods without being interrupted or distracted. Family members, colleagues at work and friends are usually very supportive once they understand what you're doing.
- It's better not to practice a relaxation exercise right after eating or when you're feeling very tired - unless of course your intention is to fall asleep.
- You'll enjoy your experience more if you choose a comfortable position in a location that is comfortably warm and not too brightly lit. Wear loose clothing and remember to remove your contact lenses or spectacles.

It's always wise to consult your health care provider before beginning the work in this book, particularly if any of the following circumstances are relevant to you:

REFLEXOLOGY REALLY WORKS by Mercedes Del Rey

- If you are over thirty or if your reaction to stress involves physical symptoms, such as frequent headaches, stomach problems, or high blood pressure. Your physician should perform a physical examination to rule out possible physical problems that may need medical attention.
- If, after starting your stress-management programme, you experience any prolonged negative physical effects, make an appointment to consult your doctor.

We're fortunate to be living in an age where your health care provider is more likely to be a helpful and supportive partner in your efforts to live a healthier life.

REFLEXOLOGY REALLY WORKS by Mercedes Del Rey

REFLEXOLOGY REALLY WORKS by Mercedes Del Rey

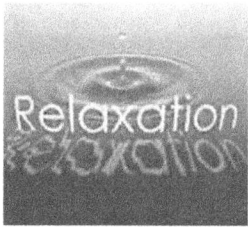

Chapter 2

Introduction to the Concept of Mindful Relaxation

Let's begin by asking ourselves what relaxation really means. In terms of technical, psychological definitions, relaxation is the emotional state of low tension, in which there is an absence of arousal that could derive from sources such as anger, anxiety, stress or fear.

In more familiar terms, relaxation is the condition where the body and mind are free from tension and anxiety. Relaxation could even be described as a mild form of ecstasy which results when the frontal lobe of the brain receives a mild chemical sedative from the rear cortex.

Most importantly, this highly desirable mental and physical condition that often seems so elusive can be acquired through meditation and the art of visualising and practising complete muscle relaxation.

Relaxation is a powerful mechanism that can improve our capacity to deal with the effects of stress. Stress in our modern, technologically advanced world is a leading cause of mental health issues and produces more than its fair share of physical problems too. So it's becoming more important than ever to learn the practical techniques of relaxation that are so beneficial for an individual's health. When we become stressed, the brain's ancient limbic system becomes more active and encourages us to behave as if we're in a fight-or-flight response mode.

As a short-term survival mechanism to save us from imminent danger, this is a fine strategy. But when the limbic system predominates, our bodies begin to suffer from the constant stress response overload and this is a very poor strategy for long term health and wellbeing. We'll be considering the limbic system in more depth shortly.

The consequences of prolonged stress have been analysed, recorded and examined for thousands of years. The modern views on the negative effects of stress on the human organism can hardly be described as new areas of exploration. We've always known that long term exposure to stress and tension can be harmful to our physical, mental and emotional wellbeing.

There have been countless answers to the challenges of stress over the long millennia of human history and modern therapies can sometimes trace their origins to ancient methods that have been successfully employed across a wide variety of cultures and civilisations. It's reassuring to know that some of these ancient methods have been successfully field-tested for thousands of years. They're as relevant today as they have always have been. And, more importantly, they work.

REFLEXOLOGY REALLY WORKS by Mercedes Del Rey

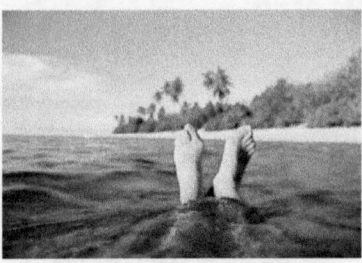

Physical relaxation techniques
One of the most neglected sources of extraordinary power in humans is the simple act of controlled breathing. The fact is that most of us hardly breathe at all, just using enough breath to sustain life but rarely straying into the realms of power that are waiting to be revealed with deeper, more controlled breathing techniques.

The breath is the essential link with life itself and our breathing reveals much about how we are feeling. The great news is that the incredibly simple breathing techniques we're about to explore are fabulously effective for reducing stress. Your body will respond instantly to the changes in oxygen uptake and the new, deeper pattern of breathing. The benefits of deeper breathing are truly extraordinary.

Natural, effective breathing techniques that incorporate deep abdominal breathing have been shown to reduce the physical symptoms of depression, anxiety and hypertension as well as neutralising the old, familiar emotional demons of anger, fear and anxiety. Just by a simple adjustment to the depth and frequency of your breathing.

We certainly owe much to the classical traditions of yoga which provide countless examples of how to bring the mind and body into complete harmony. Progressive muscle relaxation is another effective technique that requires an individual to focus on flexing and holding specific groups of muscles for a few seconds before releasing them completely.

As the individual works from the feet to the head, tensing and releasing the various muscle groups, unlocking the knots of tension and deliberately letting go of the accumulated physical stress in their bodies, they will experience a deep and powerful sense of profound relaxation. This is completely natural and an extremely beneficial product of learning to let go of all physical tension in the body.

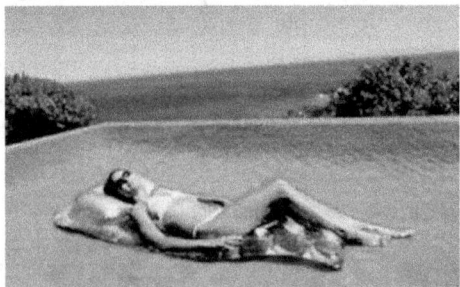

Mental Technique
The mind is the lens through which we perceive and interpret reality. Learning to bring our thoughts under gentle control bestows enormous benefits upon the practitioner. Meditation is one of the most effective methods for bringing the mind under control and for dispelling the shadows of fear, doubt and anxiety that amplify our stress responses.

Meditation has a long and celebrated history and seems to have formed a permanent and integral

REFLEXOLOGY REALLY WORKS by Mercedes Del Rey

part of the human experience since before the Stone Age. Its universal appeal has led to the development of an extraordinary variety of techniques, interpretations and disciplines amongst countless societies and civilisations. The legacy of these traditions has provided us with a richly endowed storehouse of knowledge and experience.

It is to these traditions that we turn when we consider the modern benefits of meditation. Clearly, the techniques encourage a deep, relaxed state of both mind and body and offer an insight into the inner worlds of our deeper consciousness. Meditation has been linked to measurable improvements in health and wellbeing as well as increased resistance to debilitating forces of prolonged stress.

Another helpful method, which might be described as a close parallel to meditation, is a more modern approach to stress reduction known as Hypnosis Relaxation Therapy. Professionally administered hypnosis under medical supervision has the potential to induce a profoundly deep state of relaxation.

Effective clinical hypnosis focuses on producing an altered state of consciousness under carefully controlled conditions. The therapist understands that the patient is more susceptible to suggestions in this altered state of consciousness and this creates a perfect opportunity to suggest changes in the underlying patterns of behaviour.

The technique depends very much on the skill and experience of the therapist but it's a potent method for gaining access to the subconscious programming that conditions much of our waking behaviour. Under hypnosis, the patient can be encouraged to become quite highly resistant to the effects of stress and experience a permanent increase in daily levels of calm and relaxation. The changes tend to manifest their effects very quickly so this is a fascinating potential short-cut to an improved state of relaxation.

The full potential of clinical hypnosis is still being explored but, in addition to relaxation, hypnosis therapy is being used to treat a wide variety of conditions. Treatments for conditions using hypnosis that are currently being promoted by The Mayo Clinic are; smoking addiction therapy, pain control therapy, weight loss, coping with chemotherapy, asthma, and allergy relief. This short list might represent the tip of the iceberg as further applications are explored to promote future treatments and non-invasive, prescription-free therapies.

It's sometimes quite amusing to note the latest discoveries in the field of relaxation techniques when the key methods have been quietly taught and practised for thousands of years. The important thing here is that the methods are reaching an ever widening audience as medical research reveals the benefits of these seemingly timeless methods of promoting health through relaxation.

REFLEXOLOGY REALLY WORKS by Mercedes Del Rey

Emotional Relaxation Techniques

The greatest challenge in confronting our emotional behaviour is to understand where our feelings come from. Many of us behave as if our feelings are a natural extension of our personalities. We assume that the way we feel is a perfectly natural expression of our characters. But there's a subtle clue to the origins of our behaviour in the key word 'personality'.

The *persona* was the mask worn by ancient Greek actors to portray the characters of the roles they played. Our personality is very much a product of the masks we wear, the multiple layers of learned behaviours that we acquire from our earliest childhood experiences. We rarely remember the events that shaped and imprinted our early emotional framework but their effects are often revealed in our attitudes, feelings and behaviours. Why is this relevant?

Because our behaviours do not have to be permanent features of our daily experience. They are often nothing more or less than deeply ingrained habits. Familiar habits that we resort to every day without awareness or questioning. We even defend our feelings and counter questions about our emotional reactions by stating 'Well, that's how I am!' But that is not necessarily true. Habits can change. Emotional frameworks can shift.

We are not condemned to endure one set of pre-determined negative behaviours. Cognitive behavioural therapy has amply demonstrated the effectiveness of teaching individuals to develop alternative strategies for tempering their old, knee-jerk reactions. Anger, violence, fear and destructive behaviours have been successfully tamed, reduced and transformed into wholly more appropriate actions and reactions. As you might expect, once an individual has gained control over these long-term, destructive tendencies, their lives begin to change for the better.

Emotional relaxation techniques are based on a very simple formula that identifies a moment in any situation where the individual gets to choose how they wish to feel or behave. There will be an event and there will be an outcome - usually the way you feel or react in response to the event or situation. But between those two events there is a fractional moment of inner reflection where we decide how we're going to react. This can be illustrated with a simple example. If someone asked you why you had a second head on your shoulders, you'd obviously know that their statement about you having a second head was completely wrong. It was a wildly erroneous assertion. So the statement was not even connected to you. The statement in fact revealed something about the person making the statement. Either they were suffering from some form of delusion or maybe they were just plain crazy. Either way, the statement shouldn't affect you - because it was so obviously false. But things can get a little more complicated when people make unkind assertions about your personality and - when you check your internal reference list of your good and bad qualities - you agree!

That's when you react, usually with anger, or fear or hurt. Because at some level you agree with the accusation. But what if you can learn to hesitate, to pause for a moment and think about the statement. Remember, people have an infinite number of ways to express themselves. When someone chooses to make derogatory or unkind remarks, the negativity is coming from their hearts. Not from yours.

The statement always reveals far more about the person making the statement than it ever does about the target of the comments. If someone makes an unkind comment about you and it happens to be true - what's the problem? If you know it's true, you're learning nothing new. It's entirely up to you to decide if you want to make changes to your behaviour to clean up a behavioural problem. But if someone mentions it, nothing changes. I can remember being accused in public in front of a couple of thousand people of being incredibly stupid. I congratulated the individual on working out that I was stupid because it was something I've always been aware of - so it wasn't really a surprise to me.

REFLEXOLOGY REALLY WORKS by Mercedes Del Rey

The mission is to know yourself a little more thoroughly and learn to make better choices when people make comments about you. That fractional moment is the key to catching the old reaction before it takes flight. Choosing to let go of the pre-conditioned behaviour. Learning to breathe a little more deeply. Choosing to smile as you realise that the other person really isn't talking about you at all. They're just putting their fears and phobias and prejudices on public display by advertising their in-built negativity. And that really has nothing to do with you.

You're responsible for what you feel, think, say and do. And that simple dynamic applies to pretty much everyone else too. So this is a very powerful mechanism for harnessing change at the deepest level of our behavioural framework. Learning to feel how we want to feel. Letting go of the years of pre-programmed angst, fear, anxiety and insecurity. Learning to become more of who you really are. A calmer, more creative, happier, more successful you. The you who's been waiting patiently to express themselves for most of your life.

Effects of Emotional Stress

The effects of emotional stress are different in everyone, with some people expressing different psychological signs, like irritability or depression.

Signs of emotional stress include:

- Irritability
- Depressed mood
- Anxiety
- Easily angered or frustrated
- Fatigue
- Trouble falling or staying asleep
- Loss of appetite or overeating
- Trouble concentrating
- Problems with memory
- Muscle aches
- Headaches
- Upset stomach
- Rapid heartbeat

If emotional stress lasts too long or happens too often, it can lead to more serious problems such as anxiety or depression, and physical health problems such as heart disease and obesity. According to the American Psychological Association, the majority of office visits to the doctor involve stress-related complaints.

One of the main obstacles to successful mindful relaxation is the hot-wired emotional response of the amygdala that drives us to react to stress in potentially negative ways that are not good for our health.

An unexpected but surprisingly effective method to cool down the amygdala's hot responses was developed in the seventies and has evolved into a well-researched method for dealing with a whole range of issues that effect human behaviour. The method relies on gently tapping with the fingertips on eight key areas of the body in turn.

These are areas that we instinctively touch or massage when we're stressed. These areas are

REFLEXOLOGY REALLY WORKS by Mercedes Del Rey

linked to acupressure points that can influence our behaviour. The gentle tapping reduces activity in the activity and that in turn leads to a reduction in the levels of the stress hormone, cortisol.

The real problem with stress is that it becomes such a familiar habit that we end up looking for reasons to experience it every single day. So part of the tapping technique is to identify the areas in our life that are producing the stress.

Rather than simply focusing on releasing stress, we need to find out where all the stress is coming from. In EFT, we're encouraged to score the items that are making us angry, upset, afraid or just psychologically stressed and give a mark out of ten. The higher the score, the more upset you feel about the issue. A score of zero would mean that you felt nothing about the issue.

Once you've identified the area or issue that's causing you the greatest amount of stress, you need to phrase how you feel in a simple statement. If work was the main source of tension, you could say, for example "Even though I hate my job and the constant pressure...", you then add the expression "I deeply and completely love and accept myself".

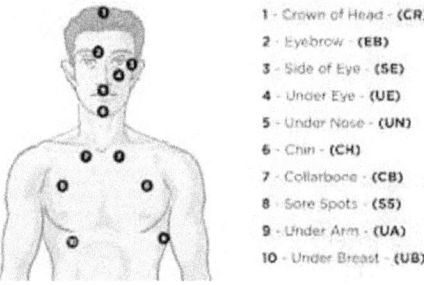

The first set of tapping is on the soft edge of the hand between the wrist and little finger. You can tap with two fingers of all your fingers and use whichever hand is most comfortable. It's great to repeat your statement at least three times before moving on to the next tapping area.

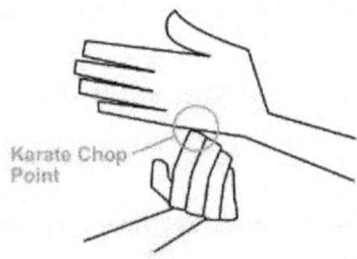

Then begin the actual process by tapping with the fingertips of both hands gently on the top of your head. Keep tapping as you repeat your original statement.

There's no limit to the number of taps or repetitions but be aware of any changes you might feel in relation to the stress source. Score the issue again. If it's the same as before, no problem.

REFLEXOLOGY REALLY WORKS by Mercedes Del Rey

Move onto the next area and keep tapping whilst you repeat the statement. Once you notice the score dropping below five, you can change your statement into a positive affirmation. "I'm feeling so much happier now that I can deal with work so much more positively".

After tapping the crown of your head, you move to your temples, close to the outer edge of your eyes, tapping once again gently as you repeat your statement.

The next point is under each eye, then under the nose, just above your upper lip.

Your chin is the next tapping point and then your hands separate to tap on your collar bone.

Then you cross your arms and tap under the armpit. The final point is just below your lowest ribs.

It's recommended that you use the technique every day for at least fifteen minutes and feel free to identify any issues that are causing you to feel stressed.

During private consultations, we've sometimes phrased emotional stress issues with the following 'set up' statement: "Even though I've had great difficulty with this issue in the past and it has caused me enormous stress and emotional discomfort - yet I deeply and completely love, respect, honour and accept myself with every part of my being".

As the issue evolves into a more positive phrasing, we modify the statement along the following lines: "I now choose deeply and completely to release and let go of all my stress and all the discomfort to become healthier and so much happier".

Your brain responds to these affirmations by re-wiring the neural connections that influence our behaviour. Tapping helps to identify the sources of stress and then reduces their influence.

The positive affirmations create the possibility of modifying our behaviour at a neural level. The result is a long-term shift in conditioned reflexes that can make a valuable contribution to effective, sustained mindful relaxation.

Once you've mastered the tapping technique, you can use it for any area of your life where you feel that change would be of benefit to you. I wholeheartedly commend the technique to you and wish you the greatest possible success with your programme and, indeed, with your life.

REFLEXOLOGY REALLY WORKS by Mercedes Del Rey

REFLEXOLOGY REALLY WORKS by Mercedes Del Rey

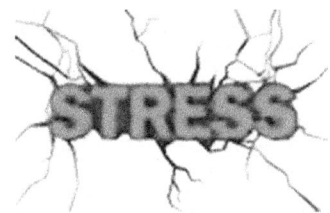

Chapter 3

How You React to Stress

The subject of stress can be quite confusing. It's such a pervasive facet of our lives that it's easy to mistake it for a natural phenomenon. But it isn't. It's time to add a measure of much-needed clarity to the subject. It is essential that we do not mistake the events around us as being the source of our stress. They are simply events. Nothing more and nothing less.

It's our conditioned reflex to our external and internal landscapes that determines whether or not we trigger the stress response. Most of us are heavily conditioned from early childhood to feel stressed under a wide variety of circumstances. Just because virtually everyone is blighted by the effects of stress and living in a world of unrelenting tension doesn't mean that the condition is in any way normal, inevitable or untreatable.

On the contrary, the good news is that our conditioned responses can be transformed so completely that life can rapidly become a much more profoundly enjoyable experience. Mastery of the stress response will be one of our most important objectives.

If you've ever had the good fortune to spend time in the presence of a great Yoga master and experienced the extraordinary calm that surrounds their every thought and action, you'll have witnessed an unforgettable demonstration of how powerful the natural state of calm can be. We're so deeply conditioned to be permanently stressed that we consider this natural expression of human potential to be an anomaly! Being overstressed – that's the anomaly.

Sources of Stress

Stress reveals itself in many different guises but most of us are typically conditioned to experience stress in response to four basic sources:

1. Environmental challenges: The list is huge and includes everything around you – such as weather, pollution, noise, traffic, crowds, the daily news on TV, family, pets and colleagues.
2. Social stressors: These are the usual, unremitting demands for your time, your energy and your attention. Family, work, social interactions and all the uncertainties and unpredictable factors of human relationships.
3. Physiological factors: Poor diet, lack of exercise, adolescence, menopause, ageing, illness, injuries and the drain of poor sleep – it's an encyclopaedic list of potential problem areas.
4. The Mental Maze: Your conditioned mental reflexes interpret the world around you according to pre-set patterns of expectation. The limbic system has been driving our survival responses since our distant ancestors first stepped down from the trees. Very handy for dealing with a hungry sabre-toothed tiger but not very helpful in developing creative, logical alternatives to life's challenges. That's precisely what the more recently evolved pre-frontal cortex is for and learning to engage its massive

capabilities is a powerful mechanism for turning down the limbic system's primitive fight or flight drives.

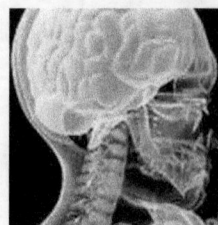

Fight-or-Flight Response
Better understanding of brain function has provided further, essential keys to explaining our behaviour and in greater depth than ever before. As you can imagine from our two million years of humanoid evolution, brain function has a long and complex history of development.

As our distant ancestors climbed down from the trees and learned to walk on two legs, they had to adapt to living on the challenging, inhospitable, grassy Savannahs of the African plains. Survival in those remote times depended very much on a part of the brain called the limbic system.

The physical and emotional responses that are driven by the limbic system are very powerful indeed and produce rapid reactions that were certainly very helpful for our early survival as a species.

We can trace reactions such as fear and anger, hunger and the sex drive to the limbic system and one part of the structure in particular exerts a powerful influence in encouraging rapid responses: we're referring to a small, almond-shaped portion of the limbic system known as the amygdala. It prompts instant reactions, particularly in the areas of fear, sexual response and hunger behaviour.

The system is primed to function from birth, prompting babies to cry when hungry and it continues to function throughout our lives, delivering emotionally-charged messages to satisfy instantly the need for pleasure and security, whilst avoiding pain and dealing with danger.

The amygdala seeks immediate reaction. It does not encourage thought, contemplation or analysis. It demands action. In a dangerous environment, it can be a life saver. In the face of a stressful situation, real or imaginary, it can be our undoing. But there's so much more to our brains than just the ancient limbic system!

If we were to identify the part of the brain that is most closely associated with the attributes of being human, it would surely be the pre-frontal cortex. This is the most highly evolved part of the brain and it's the reason that you're able to read this book.

This is the source of our creativity and imagination and provides control mechanisms for our thoughts, our feelings and our actions. This is where human flexibility is rooted. Unlike the limbic system, it develops slowly, not reaching its full capacity until our early twenties.

The pre-frontal cortex allows us to plan, to analyse, to be rational and to exercise control. Why is any of this relevant? Well, the two systems are closely linked. If the limbic system is the accelerator, putting the pedal to the metal for instant reactions, the pre-frontal cortex is the braking system, slowing things down to maintain control and seek a more logical, reasoned

REFLEXOLOGY REALLY WORKS by Mercedes Del Rey

approach. Limbic says 'Go, go, go!' Pre-frontal cortex says 'Slow down! Stop!' The Stop-Go systems work in tandem. They react together all the time in a seamless, inter-connected relationship.

As one area becomes more active, the other becomes less influential. The overwhelming need for instant action is powered by the limbic 'Go' system and this is where the stress response can move into overdrive, prompting exaggerated responses in the face of real or, most often, imagined threats and dangers.

The more we function from the limbic system, the less help we get from the highly developed pre-frontal cortex. And one of the major triggers for powering up the primordial limbic system is - stress! The more stressed you feel, the more active the limbic system becomes. And the less help you receive from the pre-frontal cortex.

So we're beginning to build a simple picture of two opposite and, in some ways, contradictory elements in the human brain. One drives us towards fear, anxiety and self-preservation.

The other enables us to delay or postpone the fear response and choose actions and behaviours that are more in tune with our long term needs and wellbeing. We know the systems are linked to each other.

We know that as one system becomes dominant, the other system powers down and reduces its capacity to influence our behaviour. And there's more. Cognitive behaviourists have another favourite term to describe the human ability for self-control and it's another potent element of the pre-frontal cortex. It's referred to as Executive Function.

EF provides us with the essential cognitive skills that give us control over our thoughts, our feelings and our actions. And the great news is that we can learn to develop Executive Function at pretty much any time in our life. Executive Function enables us to look ahead, to imagine and design plans for the future, to calculate the details and help us achieve our goals.

What a fabulous asset to have in your brain. One of our intentions is to encourage the EF to play a more dominant role in your life and take over from the limbic system's short term impulses that thrive on fear, stress and anxiety.

The stress response has been successfully measured, analysed and studied in great detail since Hans Selye (1978), the first major researcher on stress, was first able to describe what happens in the body during the fight-or-flight response. He found that any problem, imaginary or real, can cause distinct and measurable changes to the body.
As you'll probably recognise from your own direct experience of stress, these changes directly affect your heart rate, breathing rate, muscle tension, metabolism, and blood pressure. Not surprisingly, they all increase. The hands and feet become colder as blood is directed away from the extremities and from the digestive system and into the larger muscles that could be useful in assisting us to fight or run away. Some people experience butterflies in their stomachs. The pupils dilate to sharpen vision and the hearing becomes more acute.
Unfortunately, during times of repeated or chronic stress, when the fight-or-flight responses function fairly constantly without an appropriate break, other changes can be detected in the body that can produce long-term, detrimental effects on the health of the individual. The adrenal glands secrete *corticoids* (adrenaline or epinephrine, and norepinephrine), which inhibit digestion, reproduction, growth, tissue repair, and the responses of the immune and inflammatory systems.

REFLEXOLOGY REALLY WORKS by Mercedes Del Rey

To express the problem more simply, a range of essential functions that maintain physical health begin to shut down. And that's scary.

Fortunately, the same mechanism that turns the stress response on can turn it off. This is the extremely important *relaxation response*. As soon as you realise that a situation is no longer threatening and you breathe a sigh of relief, your brain stops sending emergency signals to your brain stem, which in turn ceases to send panic messages to your nervous system. Three minutes after you shut off the danger signals, the fight-or-flight response switches to neutral. Your metabolism, heart rate, breathing rate, muscle tension, and blood pressure all return to their normal, optimal levels of functioning.

REFLEXOLOGY REALLY WORKS by Mercedes Del Rey

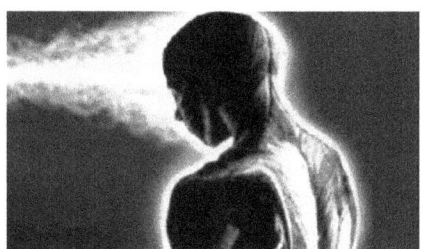

Chapter 4

Your Stress Symptoms Checklist

Chronic Stress, Physiological Imbalance and the Disease Connection

We've just examined the effects of having a surfeit of stress in our lives and there can be many causes of this unpleasant condition. Chronic or persistent stress can occur when life stressors are unrelenting. We can easily imagine the stress that flares up during a major reorganization or downsizing at work, while undergoing a messy divorce, or coping with chronic pain or disease or a life-threatening illness.

Chronic stress also takes its toll when small stressors accumulate and you are unable to recuperate from any one of them. As long as the mind perceives a threat, the body remains aroused and stressed. If your stress response remains turned on, your chances of getting a stress-related disease may be increasing dramatically.

Before you embark on your personal programme of mindful relaxation, it is helpful to consider how you're currently dealing with your stress.

Instructions: Listed below are some common ways of coping with stressful events. Mark those that most closely represent your behaviour or that you feel you use on a regular basis.

_____ 1. I ignore my own needs and just work more.
_____ 2. I seek out friends or therapists for support.
_____ 3. I eat much more than usual.
_____ 4. I engage in some type of physical exercise.
_____ 5. I get irritable and take it out on those around me.
_____ 6. I take a little time to relax, breathe, and unwind.
_____ 7. I smoke a cigarette or drink a caffeinated beverage.
_____ 8. I confront my source of stress and work to change it.
_____ 9. I withdraw emotionally
_____ 10. I change my outlook on the problem and put it in a better perspective.
_____ 11. I sleep more than I really need to.
_____ 12. I take some time off and get away from my work or the situation
_____ 13. I go out shopping and buy something to feel good.
_____ 14. I joke with my friends and use humor to feel better
_____ 15. I drink more alcohol than usual.
_____ 16. I get involved in a hobby or interest that helps me unwind
_____ 17. I take medicine to help me relax or sleep better.
_____ 18. I maintain a healthy diet.
_____ 19. I just ignore the problem and hope it will go away.
_____ 20. I pray, meditate, or enhance my spiritual life.
_____ 21. I worry about the problem but do nothing

REFLEXOLOGY REALLY WORKS by Mercedes Del Rey

_____ 22. I try to focus on the things I can control and accept the things I can't.

Evaluate your results: The even-numbered items tend to be the more constructive tactics and the odd-numbered items tend to be less constructive tactics for coping with stress. Congratulate yourself for all of the even-numbered items you checked. Think about whether you need to make some changes in your thinking or behaviour if you checked any of the odd-numbered items. Consider experimenting with some even-numbered items you haven't tried before. This workbook will assist you in making these changes.

Researchers have been looking at the relationship between stress and disease for over a hundred years. They have observed and concluded that people suffering from stress-related disorders tend to show hyperactivity in a particular "preferred system," or "stress-prone system," such as the skeletomuscular, cardiovascular, or gastrointestinal system. For example, chronic stress can result in muscle tension and fatigue for some people. For others, it can contribute to high blood pressure, migraine headaches, ulcers, or chronic diarrhoea.

Almost every system in the body can be damaged by stress. When an increase in corticoids suppresses the reproduction system, this can cause amenorrhea and failure to ovulate in women, impotency in men, and loss of libido in both.

Stress-triggered changes in the lungs increase the symptoms of asthma, bronchitis, and other respiratory conditions. Loss in insulin during the stress response may be a factor in the onset of adult diabetes. Stress suspends the body's tissue repair mechanism which, in turn, causes decalcification of the bones, osteoporosis, and susceptibility to fractures.

The inhibition of immune and inflammatory systems makes you more susceptible to colds and flu and can exacerbate some specific diseases such as cancer and AIDS. In addition, a prolonged stress response can worsen conditions such as arthritis, chronic pain, and diabetes. There are also some indications that the continued release and depletion of norepinephrine during a state of chronic stress can contribute to depression and anxiety.

The relationship between chronic stress, disease, and ageing is another fascinating area of research. Experts in ageing are examining changing patterns of disease and the increased appearance of degenerative disorders.

Over just a few generations, the threat of infectious diseases such as typhoid, pneumonia, and polio has been replaced with such "modern plagues" as cardiovascular disease, cancer, arthritis, respiratory disorders like asthma and emphysema, and a pervasive incidence of depression. As you age normally, you expect a natural slowing down of your body's functioning. But many of these mid- to late-life disorders are stress-sensitive diseases.

Currently, researchers and clinicians are asking how stress accelerates the ageing process and what can be done to counteract these pernicious and debilitating products of an over-stressed lifetime of worry and prolonged anxiety.

Check out these events and create your own schedule of recent stress experiences!

REFLEXOLOGY REALLY WORKS by Mercedes Del Rey

Event	Number 1-5	x	1 for once a month 2 for once a week 3 for once a day	=	Your Score
1. A lot more or a lot less trouble with the boss.	_____	x	_____	=	_____
2. A major change in sleeping habits (sleeping a lot more or a lot less or a change in time of day when you sleep).	_____	x	_____	=	_____
3. A major change in eating habits (eating a lot more or a lot less or very different meal hours or surroundings).	_____	x	_____	=	_____
4. A revision of personal habits (dress, manners, associations, and so on).	_____	x	_____	=	_____
5. A major change in your usual type or amount of recreation.	_____	x	_____	=	_____
6. A major change in your social activities (e.g., clubs, dancing, movies, visiting, and so on).	_____	x	_____	=	_____
7. A major change in church activities (attending a lot more or a lot less than usual).	_____	x	_____	=	_____
8. A major change in the number of family get-togethers (a lot more or a lot fewer than usual).	_____	x	_____	=	_____

REFLEXOLOGY REALLY WORKS by Mercedes Del Rey

9. A major change in your financial state (a lot worse off or a lot better off). _____ x _____ = _____

10. Trouble with in-laws. _____ x _____ = _____

11. A major change in the number of arguments with spouse (a lot more or a lot fewer than usual regarding child rearing, personal habits, and so on). _____ x _____ = _____

12. Sexual difficulties. _____ x _____ = _____

13. Major personal injury or illness _____ x _____ = _____

14. Death of a close family member (other than spouse). _____ x _____ = _____

15. Death of spouse. _____ x _____ = _____

16. Death of a close friend. _____ x _____ = _____

17. Gaining a new family member (through birth, adoption, oldster moving in, and so on). _____ x _____ = _____

18. Major change in the health or behavior of a family. _____ x _____ = _____

19. Change in residence. _____ x _____ = _____

20. Detention in jail or other institution. _____ x _____ = _____

REFLEXOLOGY REALLY WORKS by Mercedes Del Rey

21. Minor violations of the law (traffic tickets, jaywalking, disturbing the peace, and so on). _____ x _____ = _____

22. Major business readjustment (merger, reorganization, bankruptcy, and so on). _____ x _____ = _____

23. Marriage. _____ x _____ = _____

24. Divorce. _____ x _____ = _____

25. Marital separation from spouse. _____ x _____ = _____

26. Outstanding personal achievement. _____ x _____ = _____

27. Son or daughter leaving home (marriage, attending college, and so on). _____ x _____ = _____

28. Retirement from work. _____ x _____ = _____

29. Major change in working hours or conditions. _____ x _____ = _____

30. Major change in responsibilities at work (promotion, demotion, lateral transfer). _____ x _____ = _____

31. Being fired from work. _____ x _____ = _____

32. Major change in living conditions (building a new home or remodeling, deterioration of home or neighborhood). _____ x _____ = _____

33. Spouse beginning or ceasing to work outside the home.   _____ x _____ = _____

34. Taking out a mortgage or loan for a major purchase (purchasing a home or business and so on).   _____ x _____ = _____

35. Taking out a loan for a lesser purchase (a car, TV, freezer, and so on).   _____ x _____ = _____

36. Foreclosure on a mortgage or loan.   _____ x _____ = _____

37. Vacation.   _____ x _____ = _____

38. Changing to a new school.   _____ x _____ = _____

39. Changing to a different line of work.   _____ x _____ = _____

40. Beginning or ceasing formal schooling.   _____ x _____ = _____

41. Marital reconciliation with mate.   _____ x _____ = _____

42. Pregnancy.   _____ x _____ = _____

Your total score   _____ x _____ = _____

REFLEXOLOGY REALLY WORKS by Mercedes Del Rey

Scoring:
The higher your total score, the greater your risk of developing stress-related symptoms or illnesses. Of those with a score of over 100 for the past year, almost 80 percent will get sick in the near future; of those with a score of 50-100, about 50 percent will get sick in the near future; and of those with a score of 15-50, only about 30 percent will get sick in the near future. A score of less than 15 indicates that you have a low chance of becoming ill. So, the higher your score, the harder you should work to stay well.

Because individuals vary in their perception of a given life event as well as in their ability to adapt to change, we recommend that you use this standardized test only as a rough predictor of your increased risk.

Stress can be cumulative. Events from two years ago may still be affecting you now. If you think that past events may be a factor for you, repeat this test for the events of the preceding year and compare your scores.

REFLEXOLOGY REALLY WORKS by Mercedes Del Rey

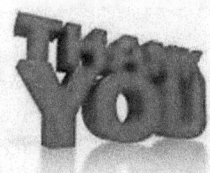

I am so delighted that you have chosen this book and it's been a pleasure writing it for you. My mission is to help as many readers as possible to benefit from the content you have just been reading. So many of us are able to take new information and apply it to our lives with really positive and long lasting consequences and it is my wish that you have been able to take value from the information I have presented.

Thank you for staying with me during this book and for reading it through to the end. I really hope that you have enjoyed the contents and that's why I appreciate your feedback so much. If you could take a couple of minutes to review the book, your views will help me to create more material that you find beneficial.

I am always delighted to hear from my readers and you can email me via the publisher at beranparry@gmail.com if you have any questions about this book or future books. Let us know how we can help you by sending a message to the same email address.

Thanks again for your support and encouragement. I really look forward to reading your review.

Stay Healthy!

REFLEXOLOGY REALLY WORKS by Mercedes Del Rey

FOR MORE BY MERCEDES DEL REY

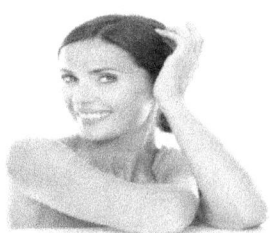

Please Visit the Web site

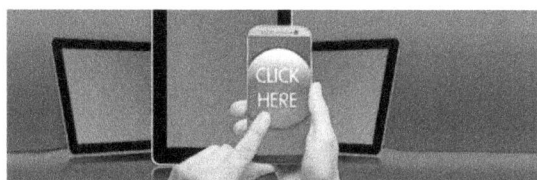

MORE FROM THE SAME PUBLISHERS
Search over the internet www.amazon.com/s/ref=dp_byline_sr_ebooks_1?ie=UTF8&field-author=Mercedes+Del+Rey&search-alias=digital-text&text=Mercedes+Del+Rey&sort=relevancerank

REFLEXOLOGY REALLY WORKS by Mercedes Del Rey

From The Same Publisher
Improve Your Immune System Naturally
(Over 50 Helpful Herbs)
Stay Well - Feel Fantastic

The more you learn about the extraordinary properties of herbs and the way they can be used to enhance your health, boost your immune system and bring relief to so many common ailments and conditions, the better your life will be

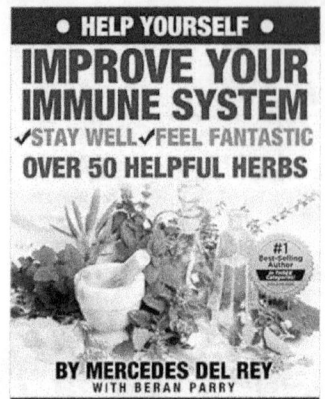

Please search this page over the internet www.amazon.com/s/ref=nb_sb_noss?url=search-alias%3Ddigital-text&field-keywords=B01BKTT8PW

REFLEXOLOGY REALLY WORKS by Mercedes Del Rey

Your Ultimate Herbal Miracle Manual
Your Permanent Handbook for Herbal Treatments
With this easy to use Herbal Miracle Manual, you will be able to:
*** Learn more about Herbs and Medicine
*** Find out how to use herbs to help some of your conditions
*** Improve your understanding of how herbs help us
*** Learn about which herbs help certain conditions
*** Broaden your understanding of the healing properties of herbs

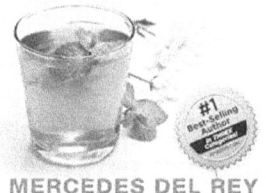

Please search this page www.amazon.com/s/ref=nb_sb_noss?url=search-alias%3Ddigital-text&field-keywords=B0185HGFVC

REFLEXOLOGY REALLY WORKS by Mercedes Del Rey

The Ultimate Herbal Detox Tea Book
(Over 75 Herbal Tea Cures for Toxic Symptoms)
Your Permanent Detox Tea Handbook

Detoxing your body was never so simple or so tasty! If you feel that your health could use a helping hand, if your wellbeing could use a boost, download your copy of the Ultimate Herbal Tea Guide right now and sip your way gently to better health and a cleaner, happier body.

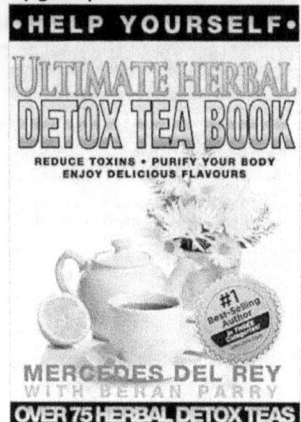

Please searc this page www.amazon.com/s/ref=nb_sb_noss?url=search-alias%3Ddigital-text&field-keywords=B019OSH1JG

www.ingramcontent.com/pod-product-compliance
Lightning Source LLC
Chambersburg PA
CBHW080722190526
45169CB00006B/2483